Department of Veterans Affairs
Health Services Research & Development Service

Evidence-based Synthesis Program

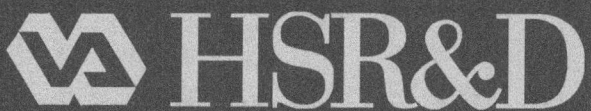

Risk Prediction Models for Hospital Readmission:
A Systematic Review

October 2011

Prepared for:
Department of Veterans Affairs
Veterans Health Administration
Health Services Research & Development Service
Washington, DC 20420

Prepared by:
Evidence-based Synthesis Program (ESP) Center
Portland VA Medical Center
Portland, OR
Devan Kansagara, M.D., M.C.R., Director

Investigators:
Principal Investigator:
Devan Kansagara, M.D., M.C.R.

Co-Investigators:
Honora Englander, M.D.
Amanda Salanitro, M.D., M.S., M.S.P.H.
David Kagen, M.D.
Cecelia Theobald, M.D.
Sunil Kripalani, M.D., M.Sc.

Research Associate:
Michele Freeman, M.P.H.

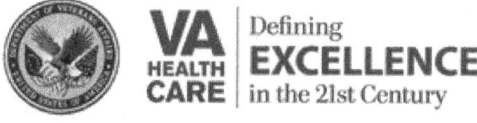

PREFACE

Health Services Research & Development Service's (HSR&D's) Evidence-based Synthesis Program (ESP) was established to provide timely and accurate syntheses of targeted healthcare topics of particular importance to Veterans Affairs (VA) managers and policymakers, as they work to improve the health and healthcare of Veterans. The ESP disseminates these reports throughout VA.

HSR&D provides funding for four ESP Centers and each Center has an active VA affiliation. The ESP Centers generate evidence syntheses on important clinical practice topics, and these reports help:

- develop clinical policies informed by evidence,
- guide the implementation of effective services to improve patient outcomes and to support VA clinical practice guidelines and performance measures, and
- set the direction for future research to address gaps in clinical knowledge.

In 2009, the ESP Coordinating Center was created to expand the capacity of HSR&D Central Office and the four ESP sites by developing and maintaining program processes. In addition, the Center established a Steering Committee comprised of HSR&D field-based investigators, VA Patient Care Services, Office of Quality and Performance, and Veterans Integrated Service Networks (VISN) Clinical Management Officers. The Steering Committee provides program oversight, guides strategic planning, coordinates dissemination activities, and develops collaborations with VA leadership to identify new ESP topics of importance to Veterans and the VA healthcare system.

Comments on this evidence report are welcome and can be sent to Nicole Floyd, ESP Coordinating Center Program Manager, at nicole.floyd@va.gov.

Recommended citation: Kansagara D, Englander H, Salanitro A, Kagen D, Theobald C, Freeman M and Kripalani S. Risk Prediction Models for Hospital Readmission: A Systematic Review. VA-ESP Project #05-225; 2011.

TABLE OF CONTENTS

EXECUTIVE SUMMARY

CONTEXT

Predicting hospital readmission risk is of great interest to identify which patients would benefit most from care transition interventions, as well as to risk-standardize readmission rates for purposes of hospital comparison.

OBJECTIVE

To summarize validated readmission risk prediction models, describe their performance, and assess suitability for clinical or administrative use.

METHODS

Data Sources: MEDLINE, CINAHL, and Cochrane Library through March 2011, EMBASE through August 2011, and hand search of reference lists.

Study Selection: Dual review to identify English language studies of prediction models tested with medical patients, with both derivation and validation cohorts.

Data extraction: Data were extracted on the population, setting, sample size, follow-up interval, readmission rate, model discrimination and calibration, type of data used, and timing of data collection.

RESULTS

Of 7,843 citations reviewed, 30 studies of 26 unique models met criteria. The most common outcome used was 30-day readmission; only one model specifically addressed preventable readmissions. Fourteen models relying on retrospective administrative data could be potentially used for standardization of readmission risk and hospital comparisons; of these, nine were tested in large US populations and had poor discriminative ability (c-statistics $0.55 - 0.65$). Seven models could potentially be used to identify high-risk patients for intervention early during a hospitalization (c-statistics $0.56 - 0.72$), and five could be used at hospital discharge (c-statistics $0.68 - 0.83$). Six studies compared different models in the same population and two of these found that functional and social variables improved model discrimination. Though most models incorporated medical comorbidity and prior utilization variables, few examined variables associated with overall health and function, illness severity, or social determinants of health.

CONCLUSIONS

Most current readmission risk prediction models, whether designed for comparative or clinical purposes, perform poorly. Though in certain settings such models may prove useful, efforts to improve their performance are needed as use becomes more widespread.

EVIDENCE REPORT

INTRODUCTION

An increasing body of literature attempts to describe and validate hospital readmission risk prediction tools. Interest in such models has grown for two reasons. First, transitional care interventions may reduce readmissions among chronically ill adults.[1-3] Readmission risk assessment could be used to help target the delivery of these resource-intensive interventions to the patients at greatest risk. Ideally, models designed for this purpose would provide clinically relevant stratification of readmission risk and give information early enough during the hospitalization to trigger a transitional care intervention, many of which involve discharge planning and begin well before hospital discharge. Second, there is interest in using readmission rates as a quality metric. Recently, the Centers for Medicare & Medicaid Services (CMS) began using readmission rate as a publicly reported metric, with plans to lower reimbursement to hospitals with excess risk-standardized readmission rates.[4] Valid risk adjustment methods are required for calculation of risk-standardized readmission rates which could, in turn, be used for hospital comparison, public reporting, and reimbursement determinations. Models designed for these purposes should have good predictive ability; be deployable in large populations; use reliable data that can be easily obtained; and use variables that are clinically related to, and validated in, the populations in which use is intended.[5]

This systematic review was performed to synthesize the available literature on validated readmission risk prediction models, describe their performance, and assess their suitability for clinical or administrative use.

METHODS

DATA SOURCES AND SEARCHES

We searched Ovid MEDLINE, CINAHL, and the Cochrane Library (Central Trial Registry, Systematic Reviews, and Abstracts of Reviews of Effectiveness) from database inception through March 2011, and EMBASE through August 2011, for English-language studies of readmission risk prediction models in medical populations. All citations were imported into an electronic database (EndNote X2, Thomson Reuters, New York, NY). Appendix A provides the search strategies in detail.

STUDY SELECTION

Seven investigators reviewed the citations and abstracts identified from electronic literature searches. Full-text articles of potentially relevant references were retrieved for further review. Each article was independently assessed by two reviewers using the eligibility criteria shown in Appendix B. Eligible articles were published in English and evaluated the ability of statistical models to predict hospital readmission risk. Because a set of predictive factors derived in only one population may lack validity and applicability,[6] we included only studies of models that were tested in both a derivation and validation cohort, even if these results were presented in separate papers. We did not pre-specify the method of validation, nor did we exclude studies in which the derivation and validation cohorts were drawn from the same population (i.e., split-half validation). We did not limit studies by diagnosis within medical populations, but we excluded studies focused on psychiatric, surgical, and pediatric populations as factors contributing to readmission risk might be considerably different in these patient groups,. Finally, we excluded studies from developing nations as these were unlikely to provide directly applicable results.

DATA EXTRACTION AND QUALITY ASSESSMENT

From each study, we abstracted the following: population characteristics, setting, number of subjects in the derivation and validation cohorts, utilization outcome, readmission rate, range of readmission rates according to predicted risk, and model discrimination. To facilitate a high-level comparison of predictor variables, we grouped final model variables into one of six categories (medical comorbidity, mental health comorbidity, illness severity, prior utilization, overall health and function, and sociodemographic/social determinants of health).[7]

To characterize the practical utility of each model, two reviewers abstracted from each study the type of data used and the timing of data collection. Disagreements between reviewers about these classifications were resolved through group discussion. Data type consisted of administrative, primary (e.g., survey, chart review), or both. Regarding timing, we classified a model as using real-time data if the variables would be available on or shortly after index hospital admission, and as using retrospective data if the variables would not be available early during a hospitalization. For example, a model using prior healthcare utilization and data from patient surveys conducted early during a hospitalization would be classified as using real-time data, while a model using index hospital length of stay or index hospital discharge diagnostic codes would be classified as using retrospective data. Because of coding delays, models relying on administrative codes from index hospital admission were considered retrospective.

We report the c-statistic, with 95% confidence interval when available, to describe model discrimination. The c-statistic, which is equivalent to the area under the receiver operating characteristic curve, is the proportion of times the model correctly discriminates a pair of high- and low-risk individuals.[8] A c-statistic of 0.5 indicates the model performs no better than chance; a c-statistic of 0.7 to 0.8 indicates modest or acceptable discriminative ability, and a threshold of greater than 0.8 indicates good discriminative ability.[9, 10] If the c-statistic was not reported, we abstracted other operational statistics such as sensitivity, specificity and predictive values for representative risk score cut-offs when available. Model calibration is the degree to which predicted rates are similar to those observed in the population. To describe model calibration we report the range of observed readmission rates from the predicted lowest to highest risk groupings.

To guide our methodologic assessment of included studies, we adapted elements – including cohort definition, follow-up, adequacy of prognostic and outcome variable measurement, and validation method – from a prognosis study quality tool and clinical decision rule assessment tool (Appendix C).[6, 11]

DATA SYNTHESIS

The included studies were too heterogenous to permit meta-analysis. Therefore, we qualitatively synthesized results, focusing on model discrimination, the populations in which the model has been tested, practical aspects of model implementation, and the types of variables included in each model.

RESULTS

From 7,843 titles and abstracts, 286 articles were selected for full-text review (Figure available as online supplement). Of these, 30 studies of 26 unique models across a broad variety of settings and patient populations met our inclusion criteria (Table 1). Most (N=23) studies were based on US healthcare data. The remainder were from Australia (2 studies), England (2), Ireland (1), Switzerland (1), or Canada (1). Fourteen studies included only patients at least 65 years of age. Of these, seven relied solely on Medicare administrative data. Four studies used VA data.

Figure 1. Risk Prediction Models for Hospital Readmission - Literature Flow

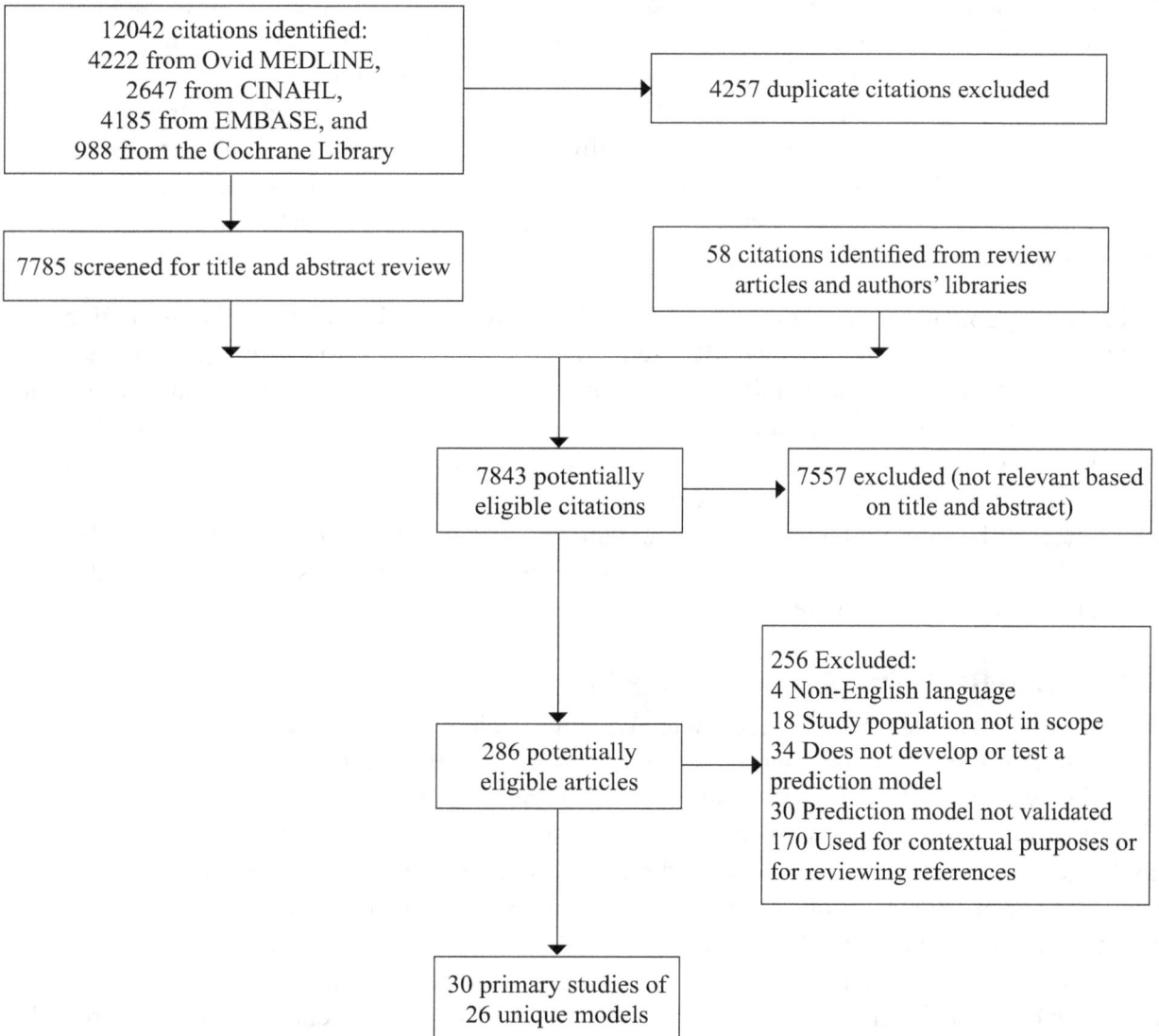

Total sample size ranged from just 173 patients to more than 2.7 million. The outcome of 30-day readmission was reported most commonly, though some models chose other follow-up intervals ranging from 14 days to 4 years. Among 21 studies reporting a c-statistic, values ranged from 0.55 – 0.83 (Table 1), but only six studies reported a c-statistic above 0.70 indicating modest discriminative ability. Performance was similar between studies using split-sample validation methods (n=21, c-statistic range 0.59-0.75), and those that used external validation methods (n=9, c-statistic range 0.53-0.83). Among models that analyzed the relationship between risk categories and actual readmission rates, a substantial gradient in readmission rate was present between patients at the lowest vs. the highest risk level. For example, among six models using 30-day readmission as an outcome, the lowest and highest risk groups differed by 20.4 to 34.5 percentage points in their actual readmission rates.

Models Relying on Retrospective Administrative Data

Fourteen models were based on retrospective administrative data and could potentially be used for hospital comparison purposes (Table 1). Most of these included medical comorbidity and prior utilization variables, but few considered mental health, functional status and social determinant variables (Table 2). The three models with c-statistics ≥ 0.70 were developed and tested in large European or Australian cohorts. One examined the risk of two or more unplanned readmissions for all hospitalized patients in England, including pediatric and obstetric patients, for one calendar year.[12] A Swiss study of potentially preventable readmissions is described in greater detail below.[13] An Australian model incorporating over 100 medical comorbidities and administrative social determinant variables performed at a modest level in asthma patients, but poorly in myocardial infarction patients.[14]

The nine large population-based or multicenter US studies generally had poor discriminative ability (c-statistics 0.55 – 0.65). The CMS used a methodologically rigorous process to create three models for congestive heart failure, acute myocardial infarction, and pneumonia admissions based on Hierarchical Condition Categories, which are groups of related comorbidities.[15-17] All three models showed relatively poor ability to predict 30-day all cause readmissions (c-statistics 0.61, 0.63, and 0.63, respectively). A recent study evaluating the CMS heart failure model, and an older heart failure model fared similarly (c-statistics 0.59 and 0.61, respectively).[18, 19] The other four US models have limited generalizability: one captured readmissions to one medical center only,[20] and the others were developed over two decades ago.[21-23]

Models Using Real-Time Administrative Data

Three administrative data-based models were designed to identify high-risk patients in real-time to potentially facilitate targeted interventions. A model with modest discriminative ability (c-statistic 0.72, 95% CI 0.70-0.75) examined 30-day heart failure readmissions in a single urban US health system with a large socioeconomically disadvantaged population.[24] It incorporated variables from an automated electronic medical record system, including numerous social factors such as number of address changes, census tract socioeconomic status, history of cocaine use, and marital status. The only study focused specifically on Medicaid enrollees used a 0 to 100 risk score for 12-month readmissions and found patient cost profiles varied widely with risk score.[25] Finally, a British model used prior utilization and comorbidity data, and also controlled for observed to expected readmission rates for the admission hospital, but predictive ability remained modest (c-statistic 0.69).[26]

Models Incorporating Primary Data Collection

Nine models incorporated survey or chart review data and could potentially be used for clinical intervention purposes, though five used data unlikely to be available early during a hospitalization. The best performing of these used administrative comorbidity and prior utilization data (c-statistic 0.77) along with functional status data (c-statistic 0.83) from the Medicare Beneficiaries Survey to predict a composite outcome of readmissions and nursing home transfers.[27] The survey was not routinely administered during index hospitalization and it is unclear to what extent the use of retrospective survey data affects the predictive ability of the model. Similarly, a medical record study in Ireland retrospectively applied a nine-item questionnaire, including items such as discharge polypharmacy, and performed modestly well (c-statistic 0.70).[28] A simple Canadian model used medical comorbidities up through index hospital discharge along with index hospital length of stay and prior utilization (c-statistic 0.68, 95%CI 0.65-0.71).[29] Increasing scores on another four-item model of medical comorbidities, prior utilization and discharge creatinine were associated with increasing readmission rates in heart failure patients.[30]

Four models incorporated primary data collected in real-time. Only two of these models have been tested in contemporary populations, the others having been conducted more than two decades ago. One survey-based model developed at six academic hospitals included social determinant, comorbidity, utilization, and self-rated health variables, but had poor predictive ability (c-statistic 0.61).[31] The Probability of Repeated Admissions (PRA) is a simple eight-item survey tool developed in older Medicare beneficiaries, but it also had poor predictive ability across several studies (c-statistic 0.56–0.61, 95% CI 0.44-0.67).[32-34]

Use of variables

A comparison of the types of variables considered for, and included in, the final models can provide some information about the contribution of different types of variables to readmission risk prediction (Table 2). Nearly all studies included medical comorbidity data and many included prior utilization variables, usually prior hospitalizations. Basic sociodemographic variables such as age and gender were considered by most studies but, in many instances, these variables did not contribute enough to be included in the final model. Table 2 also highlights important gaps in model development: few studies considered variables associated with illness severity, overall health and function, and social determinants of health.

Six studies that compared the performance of different models within the same population offer further insights about the incremental value of different types of variables (Table 3). Amarasingham and colleagues found that an automated electronic medical record-based model incorporating sociodemographic factors such as drug use and housing discontinuities, was more predictive than comorbidity-based models.[24] Coleman and colleagues found the inclusion of variables such as functional status from survey data improved model performance slightly compared to the use of utilization and comorbidity-based administrative data alone (c-statistics 0.83 vs 0.77).[27]

Other comparative studies found little difference among models. Clinical data, such as laboratory and physiologic variables, from medical records or registries did not enhance performance of claims-only CMS models.[15-17, 28] A US study of older patients found that an intricate ICD-9 code based disease complexity system added very little discriminative ability to a poorly performing Health Care Financing Authority model.[23] A large Swiss study of potentially preventable readmission risk compared a very simple non-clinical model, a Charlson comorbidity-based model, and a more complex hierarchical diagnosis and procedures based model called SQLape, finding only slight differences among them (c-statistics 0.67, 0.69, and 0.72, respectively).[13] Finally, Allaudeen and colleagues found internal medicine interns using a gestalt approach predicted readmissions with a similar poor level of ability as an older, established survey-based model (PRA) in a small, single center cohort.[34]

Potentially preventable readmissions

Only one model attempted to explicitly define and identify potentially preventable readmissions.[35] Investigators conducted a systematic medical record review to define potentially preventable readmissions and develop an administrative data-based algorithm. A subsequent publication (described above) compared the performance of three models in predicting readmissions according to their algorithm.[13]

DISCUSSION

In this systematic review, we found 26 readmission risk prediction models of medical patients tested in a variety of settings and populations. Several are being applied currently in clinical, research or policy arenas. Half the models were largely designed to facilitate calculation of risk-standardized readmission rates hospital comparison purposes. The other half were clinical models that could be used to identify high-risk patients for whom a transitional care intervention might be appropriate. Most models in both categories have poor predictive ability.

Readmission risk prediction remains a poorly understood and complex endeavor. Indeed, models of patient level factors such as medical comorbidities, basic demographic data, and clinical variables are much better able to predict mortality than readmission risk.[18, 24, 29] Broader social, environmental, and medical factors such as access to care, social support, substance abuse, and functional status contribute to readmission risk in some models, but the utility of such factors has not been widely studied.

It is likely that hospital and health system-level factors, which are not present in current readmission risk models, contribute to risk.[36] For instance, the timeliness of post-discharge follow-up, coordination of care with the primary care physician, and quality of medication reconciliation may be associated with readmission risk.[37, 38] The supply of hospital beds may independently contribute to higher readmission rates.[39] Finally, the quality of inpatient care could also contribute to risk,[40] though the evidence is mixed.[41] Though the inclusion of such hospital-level factors would conceivably improve the predictive ability of models, it would be inappropriate to include them in models that are used for risk-standardization purposes. Doing so would adjust hospital readmission rates for the very deficits in quality and efficiency that hospital comparison efforts seek to reveal, and which could be targets for quality improvement interventions.

Public reporting and financial penalties for hospitals with high 30-day readmission rates are spurring organizations to innovate and implement quality improvement programs.[42, 43] Nevertheless, the poor discriminative ability of most of the administrative models we examined raises concerns about the ability to standardize risk across hospitals in order to fairly compare hospital performance. Until risk prediction and risk adjustment become more accurate, it seems inappropriate to compare hospitals in this way and reimburse (or penalize) them on the basis of risk-standardized readmission rates. Others have reached similar conclusions,[44] and have also expressed concern that such financial penalties could exacerbate health disparities by penalizing hospitals with fewer resources.[45] Still others have argued that readmission rate is an incomplete accountability measure that fails to consider "the real outcomes of interest – health, quality of life, and value."[46]

Use of readmission rates as a quality metric assumes that readmissions are related to poor quality care and are potentially preventable. However, the preventability of readmissions remains unclear and understudied. We found only one validated prediction model that explicitly examined potentially preventable readmissions as an outcome, and it found only about one-quarter of readmissions were clearly preventable.[13] A recent systematic review of 34 studies found wide variation in the percentage of readmissions considered preventable; estimates ranged from 5% to 79%, with a median of 27%.[47] More work is needed to develop readmission risk prediction models with an outcome of preventable readmissions. This could not only improve risk-standardization efforts, but also allow hospitals to better focus limited clinical resources in readmission avoidance programs.

As with models that are used for risk-standardization, readmission risk models that are intended for clinical use also have certain requirements and limitations. Clinical models would ideally provide data prior to discharge, discriminate high- from low-risk patients, and would be adapted to the settings and populations in which they are to be used. Very few models met all these criteria, and only one of these – a single-center study – had acceptable discriminative ability.[24] As with the risk-adjustment models, most of the models developed for clinical purposes had poor predictive ability, though notable exceptions suggest the addition of social or functional variables may improve overall performance.[24, 27]

The best choice of model may depend on setting and the population being studied. The success of some models in certain populations and the lack of success of others suggest the patient-level factors associated with readmission risk may differ according to the population studied. For example, while medical comorbidities may account for a large proportion of risk in some populations, social determinants may disproportionately influence risk in socioeconomically disadvantaged populations. Our review finds, though, that very few models have incorporated such variables.

Even though the overall predictive ability of the clinical models was poor, we did find that high- and low-risk scores were associated with a clinically meaningful gradient of readmission rates. This is important given resource constraints and the need to selectively apply potentially costly care transition interventions. Even limited ability to identify a proportion of patients at risk for future high-cost utilization can increase the cost-effectiveness of such programs.[26, 48]

Of note, very few models incorporated clinically actionable data that could be used to triage patients to different types of interventions. For example, marginally housed patients, or those struggling with substance abuse, might require unique discharge services. Relatively simple, practical models that use real-time clinically actionable data, such as the Project BOOST model, have been created, but their performance has not yet been rigorously validated.[49]

Our review concurs with and adds to the findings of several other reviews that found deficiencies in the predictive abilities of risk prediction models. One recent review limited to US studies examined general risk factors for preventable readmissions, but did not search explicitly for validated models, and many of the included studies suffered from poor study design.[50] The authors suggest that, in general, measures of poor health such as comorbidity burden, prior utilization, and increasing age were associated with readmissions. Two other reviews focused on specific diagnoses and found very few readmission risk models for heart failure,[44] COPD,[51] or myocardial infarction.[52]

Our review has certain limitations. We included studies outside the United States, given that portions of US health care may resemble other countries' health systems, but applicability of models from other countries to the US may still be limited. Our classifications of data types, data collection timing, and the intended use of each model, are subject to interpretation, but we attempted to mitigate subjectivity by using a dual-review and consensus process. Finally, few studies directly compared models within the same population, and summary statistics such as the c-statistic should not be used to directly compare models across different populations.

Additional research is needed to assess the true preventability of readmissions in US health systems. Given the broad variety of factors that may contribute to preventable readmission risk, models that include factors obtained through medical record review or patient report, may be valuable. Innovations to collect broader variable types for inclusion in administrative data sets should be considered. Future studies should assess the relative contributions of different types of patient data (e.g., psychosocial factors) to readmission risk prediction by comparing the performance of models with and without these variables in a given population. These models should ideally be based on population specific conceptual frameworks of risk. Implementation of risk stratification models and their effect on work flow and resource prioritization should be assessed in a broad variety of hospital settings. Also, given that many models have limited predictive ability and may require some investment of time and cost to implement, future studies should further evaluate the relative value of clinician gestalt compared to predictive models in assessing readmission risk.

In summary, readmission risk prediction is a complex endeavor with many inherent limitations. Most models created to date, whether for hospital comparison or clinical purposes, have poor predictive ability. Though in certain settings such models may prove useful, better approaches are needed to assess hospital performance in discharging patients, as well as to identify patients at greater risk of avoidable readmission.

REFERENCES

1.   Jack BW, Chetty VK, Anthony D, et al. A reengineered hospital discharge program to decrease rehospitalization: a randomized trial. *Ann Intern Med.* Feb 3 2009;150(3):178-187.

2.   Coleman EA, Parry C, Chalmers S, et al. The care transitions intervention: results of a randomized controlled trial. *Arch Intern Med.* Sep 25 2006;166(17):1822-1828.

3.   Naylor MD, Brooten D, Campbell R, et al. Comprehensive discharge planning and home follow-up of hospitalized elders: a randomized clinical trial. *Jama.* Feb 17 1999;281(7):613-620.

4.   QualityNet. Readmission Measures Overview - Publicly reporting risk-standardized, 30-day readmission measures for AMI, HF and PN. *http://www.qualitynet.org/dcs/ContentS erver?cid=1219069855273&pagename=QnetPublic%2FPage%2FQnetTier2&c=Page.* Accessed 5/28/2011.

5.   Krumholz HM, Brindis RG, Brush JE, et al. Standards for statistical models used for public reporting of health outcomes: an American Heart Association Scientific Statement from the Quality of Care and Outcomes Research Interdisciplinary Writing Group: cosponsored by the Council on Epidemiology and Prevention and the Stroke Council. Endorsed by the American College of Cardiology Foundation. *Circulation.* Jan 24 2006;113(3):456-462.

6.   McGinn TG, Guyatt GH, Wyer PC, Naylor CD, Stiell IG, Richardson WS. Users' guides to the medical literature: XXII: how to use articles about clinical decision rules. Evidence-Based Medicine Working Group. *Jama.* Jul 5 2000;284(1):79-84.

7.   Centers for Disease Control and Prevention. Establishing a Holistic Framework to Reduce Inequities in HIV, Viral Hepatitis, STDs, and Tuberculosis in the United States *Atlanta (GA): U.S. Department of Health and Human Services, Centers for Disease Control and Prevention. October 2010. The report is available at: www.cdc.gov/socialdeterminants.*

8.   Iezzoni LI, Ed. *Risk adjustment for measuring health care outcomes. 3rd ed.* Chicago, IL: Health Administration Press; 2003.

9.   Schneeweiss S, Seeger JD, Maclure M, Wang PS, Avorn J, Glynn RJ. Performance of comorbidity scores to control for confounding in epidemiologic studies using claims data. *Am J Epidemiol.* Nov 1 2001;154(9):854-864.

10.   Ohman EM, Granger CB, Harrington RA, Lee KL. Risk stratification and therapeutic decision making in acute coronary syndromes. *Jama.* Aug 16 2000;284(7):876-878.

11.   Hayden JA, Cote P, Bombardier C. Evaluation of the quality of prognosis studies in systematic reviews. *Ann Intern Med.* Mar 21 2006;144(6):427-437.

12. Bottle A, Aylin P, Majeed A, Bottle A, Aylin P, Majeed A. Identifying patients at high risk of emergency hospital admissions: a logistic regression analysis. *J R Soc Med.* Aug 2006;99(8):406-414.

13. Halfon P, Eggli Y, Pretre-Rohrbach I, Meylan D, Marazzi A, Burnand B. Validation of the potentially avoidable hospital readmission rate as a routine indicator of the quality of hospital care. *Med Care.* Nov 2006;44(11):972-981.

14. Holman CDAJ, Preen DB, Baynham NJ, Finn JC, Semmens JB. A multipurpose comorbidity scoring system performed better than the Charlson index. *J Clin Epidemiol.* Oct 2005;58(10):1006-1014.

15. Krumholz H, Normand S, Keenan P, et al. Hospital 30-Day Heart Failure Readmission Measure: Methodology. *Report prepared for Centers for Medicare & Medicaid Services.* 2008.

16. Krumholz HM, Normand ST, Keenan PS, et al. Hospital 30-Day Acute Myocardial Infarction Readmission Measure: Methodology. *A report prepared for the Centers for Medicare & Medicaid Services.* 2008.

17. Krumholz HM, Normand ST, Keenan PS, et al. Hospital 30-Day Pneumonia Readmission Risk Measure: Methodology. *A report prepared for the Centers for Medicare & Medicaid Services.* 2008.

18. Hammill BG, Curtis LH, Fonarow GC, et al. Incremental value of clinical data beyond claims data in predicting 30-day outcomes after heart failure hospitalization. *Circulation: Cardiovascular Quality and Outcomes.* 2011;4(1):60-67.

19. Philbin EF, DiSalvo TG. Prediction of hospital readmission for heart failure: development of a simple risk score based on administrative data. *J Am Coll Cardiol.* May 1999;33(6):1560-1566.

20. Silverstein MD, Qin H, Mercer SQ, Fong J, Haydar Z. Risk factors for 30-day hospital readmission in patients <GT> or = 65 years of age. *Baylor University Medical Center Proceedings.* 2008;21(4):363-372.

21. Thomas JW. Does risk-adjusted readmission rate provide valid information on hospital quality? *Inquiry.* 1996;33(3):258-270.

22. Anderson GF, Steinberg EP. Predicting hospital readmissions in the Medicare population. *Inquiry.* 1985;22(3):251-258.

23. Naessens JM, Leibson CL, Krishan I, Ballard DJ. Contribution of a measure of disease complexity (COMPLEX) to prediction of outcome and charges among hospitalized patients. *Mayo Clin Proc.* Dec 1992;67(12):1140-1149.

24. Amarasingham R, Moore BJ, Tabak YP, et al. An automated model to identify heart failure patients at risk for 30-day readmission or death using electronic medical record data. *Med Care.* Nov 2010;48(11):981-988.

25. Billings J, Mijanovich T, Billings J, Mijanovich T. Improving the management of care for high-cost Medicaid patients. *Health Aff (Millwood)*. Nov-Dec 2007;26(6):1643-1654.

26. Billings J, Dixon J, Mijanovich T, Wennberg D. Case finding for patients at risk of readmission to hospital: development of algorithm to identify high risk patients. *Bmj*. Aug 12 2006;333(7563):327.

27. Coleman EA, Min SJ, Chomiak A, et al. Posthospital care transitions: patterns, complications, and risk identification. *Health Serv Res*. Oct 2004;39(5):1449-1465.

28. Morrissey EFR, McElnay JC, Scott M, McConnell BJ. Influence of drugs, demographics and medical history on hospital readmission of elderly patients: A predictive model. *Clinical Drug Investigation*. 2003;23(2):119-128.

29. van Walraven C, Dhalla IA, Bell C, et al. Derivation and validation of an index to predict early death or unplanned readmission after discharge from hospital to the community. *Cmaj*. Apr 6 2010;182(6):551-557.

30. Krumholz HM, Chen YT, Wang Y, Vaccarino V, Radford MJ, Horwitz RI. Predictors of readmission among elderly survivors of admission with heart failure. *Am Heart J*. Jan 2000;139(1 Pt 1):72-77.

31. Hasan O, Meltzer DO, Shaykevich SA, et al. Hospital readmission in general medicine patients: a prediction model. *J Gen Intern Med*. 2009;25(3):211-219.

32. Boult C, Dowd B, McCaffrey D, Boult L, Hernandez R, Krulewitch H. Screening elders for risk of hospital admission. *J Am Geriatr Soc*. Aug 1993;41(8):811-817.

33. Novotny NL, Anderson MA. Prediction of early readmission in medical inpatients using the Probability of Repeated Admission instrument. *Nurs Res*. Nov-Dec 2008;57(6):406-415.

34. Allaudeen N, Schnipper JL, Orav EJ, et al. Inability of providers to predict unplanned readmissions. *J Gen Intern Med*. Jul 2011;26(7):771-776.

35. Halfon P, Eggli Y, van Melle G, Chevalier J, Wasserfallen JB, Burnand B. Measuring potentially avoidable hospital readmissions. *J Clin Epidemiol*. Jun 2002;55(6):573-587.

36. Oddone EZ, Weinberger M, Horner M, et al. Classifying general medicine readmissions. Are they preventable? Veterans Affairs Cooperative Studies in Health Services Group on Primary Care and Hospital Readmissions. *J Gen Intern Med*. Oct 1996;11(10):597-607.

37. Hernandez AF, Greiner MA, Fonarow GC, et al. Relationship between early physician follow-up and 30-day readmission among Medicare beneficiaries hospitalized for heart failure. *Jama*. May 5 2010;303(17):1716-1722.

38. Kripalani S, Jackson AT, Schnipper JL, et al. Promoting effective transitions of care at hospital discharge: a review of key issues for hospitalists. *Journal of hospital medicine (Online)*. Sep 2007;2(5):314-323.

39.   Fisher E, Goodman D, Skinner J, Bronner K. Health Care Spending, Quality, and Out-
       comes - More Isn't Always Better. *The Dartmouth Institute for Health Policy & Clinical
       Practice.* 2009.

40.   Ashton CM, Wray NP. A conceptual framework for the study of early readmission as an
       indicator of quality of care. *Soc Sci Med.* Dec 1996;43(11):1533-1541.

41.   Weissman JS, Ayanian JZ, Chasan-Taber S, Sherwood MJ, Roth C, Epstein AM. Hospital
       readmissions and quality of care. *Med Care.* May 1999;37(5):490-501.

42.   Fung CH, Lim YW, Mattke S, et al. Systematic review: the evidence that publish-
       ing patient care performance data improves quality of care. *Ann Intern Med.* Jan 15
       2008;148(2):111-123.

43.   The Care Transitions Quality Improvement Organization Support Center (QIOSC). http://
       www.cfmc.org/caretransitions. *Accessed 6/1/11.*

44.   Ross JS, Mulvey GK, Stauffer B, et al. Statistical models and patient predic-
       tors of readmission for heart failure: a systematic review. *Arch Intern Med.* Jul 14
       2008;168(13):1371-1386.

45.   Joynt KE, Jha AK. Who has higher readmission rates for heart failure, and why? Implica-
       tions for efforts to improve care using financial incentives. *Circulation: Cardiovascular
       Quality and Outcomes.* 2011;4(1):53-59.

46.   Axon RN, Williams MV, Axon RN, Williams MV. Hospital readmission as an account-
       ability measure. *Jama.* Feb 2 2011;305(5):504-505.

47.   van Walraven C, Bennett C, Jennings A, et al. Proportion of hospital readmissions
       deemed avoidable: a systematic review. *Cmaj.* Apr 19 2011;183(7):E391-402.

48.   Mukamel DB, Chou CC, Zimmer JG, Rothenberg BM. The effect of accurate patient
       screening on the cost-effectiveness of case management programs. *Gerontologist.* Dec
       1997;37(6):777-784.

49.   Society of Hospital Medicine Project Boost Better Outcomes for Older Adults through
       Safe Transitions. Tool for Addressing Risk: A Geriatric Evaluation for Transitions. *http://
       www.hospitalmedicine.org/ResourceRoomRedesign/RR_CareTransitions/PDFs/TAR-
       GET_screen_v22.pdf.* Accessed 5/28/11.

50.   Vest JR, Gamm LD, Oxford BA, et al. Determinants of preventable readmissions in the
       United States: a systematic review. *Implement Sci.* 2010;5:88.

51.   Bahadori K, FitzGerald JM. Risk factors of hospitalization and readmission of pa-
       tients with COPD exacerbation--systematic review. *Int J Chron Obstruct Pulmon Dis.*
       2007;2(3):241-251.

52.   Desai MM, Stauffer BD, Feringa HHH, Schreiner GC. Statistical models and patient pre-
       dictors of readmission for acute myocardial infarction: a systematic review. *Circulation.*
       Sep 2009;Cardiovascular Quality & Outcomes. 2(5):500-507.

53.   Holloway JJ, Medendorp SV, Bromberg J. Risk factors for early readmission among veterans. *Health Serv Res.* Apr 1990;25(1 Pt 2):213-237.

54.   Howell S, Coory M, Martin J, et al. Using routine inpatient data to identify patients at risk of hospital readmission. *BMC Health Serv Res.* 2009;9:96.

55.   Smith DM, Norton JA, McDonald CJ. Nonelective readmissions of medical patients. *J Chronic Dis.* 1985;38(3):213-224.

56.   Smith DM, Weinberger M, Katz BP, Moore PS. Postdischarge care and readmissions. *Med Care.* Jul 1988;26(7):699-708.

57.   Smith DM, Katz BP, Huster GA, Fitzgerald JF, Martin DK, Freedman JA. Risk factors for nonelective hospital readmissions. *J Gen Intern Med.* Dec 1996;11(12):762-764.

58.   Burns R, Nichols LO. Factors predicting readmission of older general medicine patients. *J Gen Intern Med.* Sep-Oct 1991;6(5):389-393.

59.   Evans RL, Hendricks RD, Lawrence KV, Bishop DS. Identifying factors associated with health care use: a hospital-based risk screening index. *Soc Sci Med.* 1988;27(9):947-954.

60.   Charlson ME, Pompei P, Ales KL, MacKenzie CR. A new method of classifying prognostic comorbidity in longitudinal studies: development and validation. *J Chronic Dis.* 1987;40(5):373-383.

61.   Eggli Y. [Pre´vision des couˆts hospitaliers fonde´s sur le profil des patients] Hospital costs prevision grounded on case-mix. *Chardonne, Switzerland: SQLape sa`rl.* 2005.

62.   Tabak YP, Johannes RS, Silber JH, Tabak YP, Johannes RS, Silber JH. Using automated clinical data for risk adjustment: development and validation of six disease-specific mortality predictive models for pay-for-performance. *Med Care.* Aug 2007;45(8):789-805.

63.   Bowen OR, Roper WL. Medicare Hospital Mortality Information, 1987. Region IX: American Samoa, Arizona, Guam, Hawaii, Nevada. Publication No. HCFA 00651. Washington, DC, US Government Printing Office, 1988.

TABLE 1.   Characteristics of validated readmission risk prediction models

Study	Population	Setting	No. of patients, derivation cohort	No. of patients, validation cohort*	Utilization outcome†	Actual readmission rate (% of patients)		Range of readmission rates according to predicted risk (validation cohort)	Model discrimination (c-statistic‡ unless specified otherwise)
						Derivation cohort	Validation cohort		
Models relying on retrospective administrative data									
Anderson, 1985[22]	Medicare patients (excluded ESRD pts), 1974-1977	US, general population	21043	10522	60-day readmissions	NR	NR	4 – 40 (lowest to highest decile)§	NR
Bottle, 2006[12]	Inpatients, 2000-2001	England, general population	~1373755||	~1373754||	12-month readmissions	9.80 overall		---	All patients: 0.72 Patients with ambulatory care sensitive conditions¶: 0.75 All patients (12 month deaths excluded): 0.70
CMS model, AMI Krumholz 2008[16]	Medicare AMI patients ≥ 65 yr, 2005-2006	US, general population	100465	100285	30-day readmissions	18.9	19.2	8. 0 – 33.0 (lowest to highest decile)	0.63
CMS model, CHF Krumholz, 2008[15]	Medicare CHF patients ≥ 65 yr, 2003-2004	US, general population	283919	283528	30-day readmissions	23.6	23.7	15.0 - 37.0 (lowest to highest decile	0.6
CMS model, Pneumonia Krumholz, 2008[17]	Medicare pneumonia patients ≥ 65 yr, 2005-2006	US, general population	226545	226706	30-day readmissions	17.4	17.5	9.0 – 31.0 (lowest to highest decile)	0.63
Halfon, 2006[13]	All hospitalizations in year 2000	Switzerland, general population	65740	66069	30-day potentially avoidable readmissions	5.1	5.2	---	Nonclinical: 0.67 Charleson based: 0.69 SQLape: 0.72
Hammill, 2011[18]	CHF registry patients ≥ 65 yr, 2004-2006	US. general population	24163#		30-day readmissions	21.9 overall		Claims-only: 14.4 – 32.7 (lowest to highest decile) Claims-clinical: 13.5 – 33.9	Claims-only: 0.59 Claims-clinical: 0.60
Holloway, 1990[53]	Medical, neurologic, surgical, and geriatric inpatients, 1981-1982	US, single VA hospital	2970	unclear	30-day readmissions	22.0 overall		---	NR

Risk Prediction Models for Hospital Readmission: A Systematic Review

Study	Population	Setting	No. of patients, derivation cohort	No. of patients, validation cohort*	Utilization outcome†	Actual readmission rate (% of patients)		Range of readmission rates according to predicted risk (validation cohort)	Model discrimination (c-statistic‡ unless specified otherwise)
						Derivation cohort	Validation cohort		
Holman, 2005[14]	Medical, surgical, psychiatric inpatients, 1989-1997	Western Australia, general population	326,456	5289 (asthma) 5265 (AMI)	30-day readmissions	NR	NR	---	Asthma 0.71 AMI 0.64
Howell, 2009[54]	General medical inpatients with ambulatory care sensitive condition¶ 2005-2006	Queensland, Australia, general population	13207	4492	12-month readmissions	45.5	45.1	LR+ readmission for risk scores 50, 70, 80: 2.04, 3.11, 7.02 (overall range 0 – 100)	0.65
Naessens, 1992[23]	Inpatients ≥ 65 yr, 1980, 1985, and 1987	US, general population in a single county	5854	randomly selected10% of derivation cohort	60-day mortality/ readmissions	20.8 overall		15.6 – 36.0 (lowest to highest quartile)	HCFA alone 0.59 (SE=0.01) HCFA + COMPLEX 0.61 (SE=0.01)
Philbin, 1999[19]	CHF inpatients, 1995	US, multicenter in a single state	21227	21504	CHF readmissions within calendar year	21.3 overall		9.8 – 45.4 (lowest to highest ninth)	Simple scoring system: 0.60 Weighted scoring system: 0.61
Silverstein, 2008[20]	Inpatients ≥ 65 yr, 2002-2004	US, multicenter in a single city	19528	9764	30-day readmissions	11.7 overall		---	0.65 (same for both Elixhauser and HRDES methods)
Thomas, 1996[21]	Medicare inpatients ≥ 65 yr, 1989-1991	US, multicenter in a single state	12 different cohorts based on diagnosis; range 1163-14590		15-, 30-, 60-, and 90-day readmissions	3 - 40** overall		---	among 8 medical conditions and 4 time periods, c statistic ranged from 0.55-0.61
Models using administrative data in real time									
Amarasingham, 2010[24]	CHF patients, 2007-2008	US, single center	1029	343	30-day readmissions	24.1 overall		12.2 – 45.7 (lowest to highest quintile)	0.72 (0.70-0.75)
Billings, 2007[25]	Patients eligible for mandatory Medicaid managed care enrollment, 2000-2004	US, general population in a single city	~35000‖	~35000‖	12-month readmissions	NR	NR	NR (inpatient costs ranged 23,687 – 44,385 for risk scores 50-90, overall range 0 - 100)	Risk scores range 0-100 Using risk score 50+, Sens 58%, Spec 74%, PPV 69.5%, LR+ 2.23

Study	Population	Setting	No. of patients, derivation cohort	No. of patients, validation cohort*	Utilization outcome†	Actual readmission rate (% of patients) Derivation cohort	Actual readmission rate (% of patients) Validation cohort	Range of readmission rates according to predicted risk (validation cohort)	Model discrimination (c-statistic‡ unless specified otherwise)
PARR model Billings, 2006[26]	Inpatients with an ambulatory care sensitive reference condition¶ 2002-2003	England, general population	10% of hospital episodes for all England	A second 10% sample of hospital episodes for all England	12-month readmissions	NR	NR	---	0.69
Models using retrospective primary data collection									
Coleman, 2004[27]	Medicare inpatients ≥ 65 yr, 1997-1998	US, general population	700	704	30-day "complicated care transitions"††	21.9	25.0	---	administrative data model: 0.77 administrative + self-report data: 0.83
Krumholz, 2000[30]	Medicare CHF patients ≥ 65 yr, 1994-1995	US, multicenter in a single state	1129	1047	180-day readmissions	50.0	47.0	All-cause: 26.0 – 59.0 CHF: 9.0 – 31.0 (lowest to highest tertile)	Number of risk factors associated with readmission risk (P<0.0001). 0 risk factors: 26% 3-4 risk factors: 59%
Morrissey, 2003[28]	Medical inpatients ≥ 65 yr, 1997-1998	Ireland, single rural hospital	487	732	12-month readmissions	40.7	29.0	---	0.70
Smith Index (original) Smith, 1985[55]	Medical inpatients, 1979-1980	US, single county hospital	1007	499	90-day readmissions	16.9	NA	7.3 – 38.0 (lowest to highest octile)	Sens 59.0%, Spec 69.3%, PPV 29.9% LR+ 1.92
Smith Index validation Smith, 1988[56]	Medical inpatients, 1985	US, single county hospital	502 (control) 499 (intervention)		Readmissions/ month/patient (mean 180 days f/u)	NA	10.0	0.07 – 0.18 (lowest to highest tertile)	NR
Smith Index validation Smith, 1996[57]	Medical inpatients ≥ 45 yr, 1988-1990	US, single VA hospital		662 (validation)	90-day readmissions	NA	20.1	---	0.66
Van Walraven, 2010[29]	Medical and surgical inpatients	Canada, multicenter	4812 patients — split derivation/ internal validation	1M patients from Discharge Abstract Database for external validation	30-day readmissions	7.3	7.3	0 – 42.9 (scores 0 – 17, footnote – corresponding to expected probability of readmission/death of 2.0 – 34.6%)	0.68 (0.65-0.71)
Models using primary data collected in real time									
Burns, 1991[58]	Medical inpatients ≥ 65 yr, 1987	US, single VA hospital	134	34	60-day readmissions	30.6 overall		---	NR

Risk Prediction Models for Hospital Readmission: A Systematic Review

Study	Population	Setting	No. of patients, derivation cohort	No. of patients, validation cohort*	Utilization outcome†	Actual readmission rate (% of patients)		Range of readmission rates according to predicted risk (validation cohort)	Model discrimination (c-statistic‡ unless specified otherwise)
						Derivation cohort	Validation cohort		
Evans, 1988[59]	Medical, neurologic, and surgical inpatients over a 6 week period	US, single VA hospital	532	177	Composite of 60-day readmission, nursing home placement, or LOS longer than expected per mean LOS of DRG	21.0 overall (60-day readmissions)		% high-care users: 34.7 – 91.7 (lowest to highest eighth)	Risk score range 0-8; Score >= 3: Sens 0.60, Spec 0.76, LR+ 2.5; Score >= 4: Sens 0.42, Spec 0.93, LR+ 6
Hasan, 2009[31]	Medical inpatients, 2001-2003	US, multicenter	7287	3659	30-day readmissions	17.5	17.4	5.9 – 28.9 (lowest to highest quartile)	0.61
PRA (original) Boult, 1993[32]	Non-institutionalized Medicare patients ≥ 70 yr, 1984	US, general population	2942	2934	4 year readmissions	28.4	NA	26.1 (score 0-3) – 41.8 (score 4+)	0.61 (SE=0.01)
PRA validation Allaudeen, 2011[34]	Medical inpatients ≥ 65 yr, 5 week period in 2008	US, single academic center	NA	159	30-day readmissions	NA	32.7	---	PRA 0.56 (0.44-0.67); Prediction by physician 0.58-0.59 (0.46-0.70); Prediction by non-physician provider 0.50-0.55 (0.38 – 0.67)
PRA validation Novotny, 2008[33]	Medical inpatients, 2005-2007	US, single academic center	1077	NA	41-day readmissions	NA	14.0	---	PRA score 0.53 cutpoint, LR+ 1.67

Abbreviations: DRG denotes Diagnosis Related Group; LR+, Positive Likelihood Ratio; NA, Not Applicable; NR, Not Reported; PARR, Patients at Risk for Re-hospitalization algorithm; PRA, Probability of Repeated Admissions; SE, Standard Error.

* The most recent validation cohort is listed if a study had multiple validation cohorts.

† Unplanned, all-cause readmissions unless otherwise specified

‡ Validation cohort values for the c-statistic are listed if a study provided c-statistic values for both validation and derivation cohorts. 95% confidence interval is provided in parentheses, if reported.

§ Approximate values of data presented in a bar graph.

‖ The total number of subjects was divided equally between the derivation and validation cohorts, but the exact numbers were not specified.

¶ Reference conditions such as congestive heart failure, chronic obstructive pulmonary disease, diabetes, and asthma, for which timely and effective case-management has the potential to reduce the risks of readmission.

Used bootstrap method for internal validation, no separate validation cohort

** Reports 15-, 30-, 60-, and 90-day readmission rates for 12 different conditions

†† At least one transfer from lower to higher intensity care environment

TABLE 2.   Variables considered by studies in evaluating the risk of readmission

Variable	Included in final model in (N) studies	Evaluated but not included in (N) studies	Not considered* in (N) studies
Medical comorbidities			
Specific diagnoses or comorbidity index	(24) 12-21, 23, 25-32, 53, 54, 57-59	(0)	(3) 22, 24, 55
Mental health comorbidities			
Mental illness	(9) 13-15, 17, 18, 24, 25, 54, 59	(4) 16, 20, 26, 58	(11) 19, 22, 23, 28-32, 53, 55, 57
EtOH/substance use	(11) 13-15, 17-19, 24-26, 53, 54	(5) 16, 20, 28, 57, 59	(8) 22, 23, 29-32, 55, 58
Illness severity			
Illness severity index	(1) 24	(1) 58	(19) 12, 13, 15-18, 20, 23, 26, 28-32, 53-55, 57, 59
Lab findings	(4) 18, 30, 55, 57	(1) 28	(15) 12, 13, 15-17, 20, 23, 26, 29, 31, 32, 53, 54, 58, 59
Other†	(4) 2, 3, 20, 2	(4) 18, 30, 57, 59	(11) 15-17, 20, 26, 28, 29, 31, 32, 54, 55
Prior utilization			
Hospitalizations	(14) 12, 13, 22, 24-28, 30-32, 54, 58, 59	(1) 29	(10) 15-20, 23, 53, 55, 57
ER visits	(4) 25, 29, 55, 57	(1) 24	(17) 15-20, 22, 23, 26, 28, 30-32, 53, 54, 58, 59
Clinic visits/ Missed clinic visits	(3) 24, 25, 32	(0)	(19) 15-20, 22, 23, 26, 28-31, 53-55, 57-59
Index hospital length of stay	(4) 19, 21, 29, 31	(3) 30, 53, 58	(15) 15-18, 20, 22-24, 26, 28, 32, 54, 55, 57, 59
Overall health and function			
Functional status; ADL dependence; mobility	(2) 27, 57	(6) 29-32, 58, 59	(14) 15-20, 22-24, 26, 28, 53-55
Self-rated health, quality of life	(3) 27, 31, 32	(2) 28, 57	(17) 15-20, 22-24, 26, 29, 30, 53-55, 58, 59
Cognitive impairment	(7) 15-18, 28, 57, 59	(5) 20, 31, 32, 54, 58	(9) 19, 22-24, 26, 29, 30, 53, 55
Visual or hearing impairment	(1) 27	(1) 32	(21) 15-20, 22-24, 26, 28-32, 53-55, 57-59

Variable	Included in final model in (N) studies	Evaluated but not included in (N) studies	Not considered* in (N) studies
Sociodemographic factors			
Age	(19) 12-18, 20-23, 25-27, 32, 53, 54, 57, 59	(7) 19, 24, 29-31, 55, 58	(1) 28
Gender	(15) 12-18, 20-26, 32	(8) 19, 29-31, 53-55, 58	(1) 28
Race/ethnicity	(7) 12, 14, 19, 20, 22, 25, 26	(8) 24, 30-32, 54, 55, 57, 58	(8) 15-18, 23, 28, 29, 53
Social determinants of health			
SES/income/employment status	(5) 12, 14, 24, 25, 54	(7) 20, 26, 31, 32, 57-59	(10) 15-19, 22, 23, 28, 29, 53
Insurance status‡	(6) 19, 20, 24, 27, 31, 53	(1) 57	(5) 30, 32, 55, 58, 59
Education	(0)	(4) 28, 31, 32, 58	(17) 15-20, 22-24, 26, 29, 30, 53-55, 57, 59
Marital status/# of people in home	(4) 24, 28, 31, 59	(6) 29, 32, 53, 54, 57, 58	(11) 15-20, 22, 23, 26, 30, 55
Caregiver availability, other social support	(2) 32, 57	(1) 31	(19) 15-20, 22-24, 26, 28-30, 53-55, 57-59
Access to care/rurality	(5) 19, 22, 31, 53, 54	(2) 20, 29	(14) 15-18, 23, 24, 26, 28, 30, 32, 55, 57-59
Discharge location (home, NH)	(2) 19, 20	(1) 53	(18) 15-18, 22-24, 26, 28-32, 54, 55, 57-59

Six studies did not report candidate variables and only reported the final model.[12-14, 21, 25, 27]

† Examples include use of telemetry, shock, planned vs emergent index hospitalization, heart rate, ejection fraction.

‡ This category is not relevant to studies of Medicare patients[15-18, 23] and non-US studies.[12, 13, 28, 29, 54]

TABLE 3.   Studies that compared models within a population

Study and models compared	Model description	C-statistic (95% CI or SE if reported)
Halfon, 2006[13]		
Nonclinical model	Age, sex, prior utilization	0.67
Modified Charlson score based model	Charlson score[60] plus prior utilization	0.69
Modified SQLape model[61]	Complex administrative model combining comorbidity, age, and utilization data into 49 risk categories	0.72
Hammill 2011[18]		
Claims-only model	CMS administrative heart failure model[15]	0.59
Claims-clinical model	CMS heart failure model + serum creatinine, serum sodium, hemoglobin, systolic blood pressure	0.60
Allaudeen, 2011[34]		
PRA*[32]	Age, sex, self-rated health, availability of informal caregiver, coronary disease, diabetes, hospital admission within past year, prior utilization	0.56 (0.44-0.67)
Prediction by physician	Interns, residents, and attending physicians predicted chance of readmission based on overall evaluation of patient	0.58-0.59 (0.46-0.70)
Prediction by non-physician provider	Nurses and case managers predicted chance of readmission based on overall evaluation of patient	0.50-0.55 (0.38-0.67)
Amarasingham, 2010[24]		
ADHERE mortality model	Blood urea nitrogen, creatinine, and systolic blood pressure	0.56 (0.54-0.59)
CMS heart failure model[15]	Complex administrative comorbidity model consisting of age, sex, and 35 hierarchical condition categories	0.66 (0.63-0.68)
Tabak mortality model[62]	Age, 17 lab and vital sign variables within 24 hours of hospital presentation	0.61 (0.59-0.64)
Electronic readmission model	Includes Tabak mortality score, history of depression or anxiety, single status, sex, residential stability, Medicare status, residence census tract in lowest socioeconomic quintile, history of confirmed cocaine use, history of missed clinic visit, use of a health system pharmacy, number of prior admissions, presented to emergency department between 6 am and 6 pm for index admission.	0.72 (0.70-0.75)

Coleman, 2004[27]		
Administrative model	Age, sex, prior utilization, Medicaid status, Charlson score,[60] heart disease, cancer, diabetes	0.77
Administrative + self-report model	Administrative model + self-rated health, ADL assistance need, visual impairment, functional status	0.83
Naessens, 1992[23]		
Modified Health Care Financing Administration (HCFA) mortality model[63]	Age, sex, 16 DRG, and 8 comorbidities	0.59 (SE=0.01)
HCFA + COMPLEX	Complicated administrative model incorporating DRG based disease staging and number of body systems affected + HCFA	0.61 (SE=0.01)

Abbreviations: ADHERE denotes Acute Decompensated Heart Failure Registry; CI, Confidence Interval; CMS, Center for Medicaid and Medicare Services; COMPLEX, a measurement of comorbidity and disease severity;[23] HCFA, Health Care Financing Administration; IDI, Integrated Discrimination Improvement; PRA, Probability of Repeated Admission; SE, Standard Error.

* Variables were obtained from chart abstraction, whereas original PRA instrument is based on patient surveys.

APPENDIX A. SEARCH STRATEGY

Databases: Ovid Medline(R) 1996 to June 3 2010/Ovid Medline(R) and Ovid OLDMEDLINE(r) 1948 to June Week 3 2010/Ovid MEDLINE(R) In-Process & Other Non-Indexed Citations

Initial search: June 24, 2010

Update search: March 31, 2011

#	Searches	Results
1	exp Patient Readmission/	5473
2	readmi$.mp.	12202
3	rehosp$.mp.	2507
4	1 or 2 or 3	13761
5	exp Risk/	620133
6	model$.mp.	1748945
7	predict$.mp.	693749
8	risk$.mp.	1163956
9	util$.mp.	380641
10	5 or 6 or 7 or 8 or 9	3398624
11	4 and 10	5897
12	"smith index".mp.	3
13	"Probability of Repeated Admissions".mp.	1
14	11 or 12 or 13	5901
15	limit 14 to "all adult (19 plus years)"	4095
16	remove duplicates from 15	4001
	Update search additional yield	558

Databases: Cochrane Central Trial Registry (CCTR)/Cochrane Database of Systematic Reviews (CDSR)/Database of Abstracts of Reviews of Effectiveness (DARE)

Searched: June 24, 2010

Update search: March 31, 2011

#	Searches	Results
1	exp Patient Readmission/	401
2	readmi$.mp.	1478
3	rehosp$.mp.	523
4	1 or 2 or 3	1857
5	exp Risk/	18547
6	model$.mp.	37010
7	predict$.mp.	28433
8	risk$.mp.	63301
9	util$.mp.	13015
10	5 or 6 or 7 or 8 or 9	112650
11	4 and 10	975
12	"smith index".mp.	0
13	"Probability of Repeated Admissions".mp.	0
14	11 or 12 or 13	975
	After deduplication with previous search 960 unique citations	
	Update search additional yield: 137	

Database: EMBASE

Date: August 29, 2011

#	Searches	Results
1	'hospital readmission'/exp	7,965
2	readmi* AND [embase]/lim	13,680
3	rehosp* AND [embase]/lim	2,913
4	#1 OR #2 OR #3	17,205
5	'risk'/exp	1,050,898
6	model* AND [embase]/lim	1,786,265
7	predict* AND [embase]/lim	920,849
8	risk* AND [embase]/lim	1,496,969
9	util* AND [embase]/lim	502,028
10	#5 OR #6 OR #7 OR #8 OR #9	4,175,899
11	#4 AND #10	7,846
12	'smith index' AND [embase]/lim	3
13	'probability of repeated admissions'	1
14	#11 OR #12 OR #13	7,850
15	#11 OR #12 OR #13 AND ([adult]/lim OR [aged]/lim)	4,185

after deduplication with previous searches 1358 unique citations

Database: CINAHL Plus with Full Text 1986 - 2010

Initial search: June 24, 2010

Update search: March 31, 2011

Search ID#	Search Terms	Search Options	Results
S21	#S16 NOT #S20	Search modes - Boolean/Phrase	122
S20	S13 or S14 or S18	Narrow by SubjectAge3: - Aged, 80 and over Narrow by SubjectAge2: - Adult: 19-44 years Narrow by SubjectAge1: - Middle Aged: 45-64 years Narrow by SubjectAge0: - Aged: 65+ years Search modes - Boolean/Phrase	1024
S19	S13 or S14 or S18	Search modes - Boolean/Phrase	1789
S18	S11 and S17	Search modes - Boolean/Phrase	1789
S17	S1 or S2	Search modes - Boolean/Phrase	3606
S16	S12 or S13 or S14	Narrow by SubjectAge3: - Aged, 80 and over Narrow by SubjectAge2: - Adult: 19-44 years Narrow by SubjectAge1: - Middle Aged: 45-64 years Narrow by SubjectAge0: - Aged: 65+ years Search modes - Boolean/Phrase	1146
S15	S12 or S13 or S14	Search modes - Boolean/Phrase	2013
S14	"probability of repeated admissions"	Limiters - Published Date from: 19860101-20100631 Search modes - Boolean/Phrase	1

Search ID#	Search Terms	Search Options	Results
S13	"smith index"	Limiters - Published Date from: 19860101-20100631 Search modes - Boolean/Phrase	0
S12	S4 and S11	Search modes - Boolean/Phrase	2013
S11	S5 or S6 or S7 or S8 or S9 or S10	Search modes - Boolean/Phrase	501973
S10	util*	Limiters - Published Date from: 19860101-20100631 Search modes - Boolean/Phrase	108769
S9	risk*	Limiters - Published Date from: 19860101-20100631 Search modes - Boolean/Phrase	259597
S8	predict*	Limiters - Published Date from: 19860101-20100631 Search modes - Boolean/Phrase	87796
S7	"model*"	Limiters - Published Date from: 19860101-20100631 Search modes - Boolean/Phrase	149297
S6	(MH "Risk Factors")	Limiters - Published Date from: 19860101-20100631 Search modes - Boolean/Phrase	55640
S5	(MH "Risk Assessment")	Limiters - Published Date from: 19860101-20100631 Search modes - Boolean/Phrase	27742
S4	S1 or S2 or S3	Search modes - Boolean/Phrase	3959
S3	rehosp*	Limiters - Published Date from: 19860101-20100631 Search modes - Boolean/Phrase	684
S2	readmi*	Limiters - Published Date from: 19860101-20100631 Search modes - Boolean/Phrase	3606
S1	(MH "Readmission")	Limiters - Published Date from: 19860101-20100631 Search modes - Boolean /Phrase	2514
Update search additional yield			122

APPENDIX B. INCLUSION/EXCLUSION CRITERIA FOR REVIEW OF FULL-TEXT ARTICLES

1. Is the full text of the article in English?
   Yes ....Proceed to #2
   No .... Code **X1**. STOP

2. Does the study population include adult patients admitted to a medical service?
   Yes ....Proceed to #3
   No .... Code **X2**. STOP

3. Is the article a primary study that develops or tests prediction models for risk of hospital readmission?
   Yes .... Proceed to #4
   No ....Code **X3**. Proceed to #5

4. Is the model tested in both a derivation and validation cohort, or is it a validation of a previously developed model?
   Yes .... Code **I4**. Proceed to #6
   No ....Code **X4**. Proceed to #6

5. Is the article a systematic review or meta-analysis of prediction models for risk of hospital readmission?
   Yes ....Code **X5**. Proceed to #6
   (Eligible primary studies identified in systematic reviews will be coded I4).

   No .... Proceed to #6

6. If article meets none of the above criteria but may be useful for background/discussion, add code "B."

Population: Adult patients admitted to a medical service. Post-surgical patients and psychiatric re-admissions are excluded.

Intervention: Risk prediction models derived and validated in a cohort of medical inpatients.

Comparator: Studies comparing the performance of two or more risk prediction models in a population will be included.

Outcomes: Hospital readmission – including all-cause readmissions, condition-specific readmissions, and potentially preventable readmissions. Readmission of inpatients to ICU is excluded.

Timing: No restrictions.

Setting: Exclude studies conducted in health systems of developing nations.

APPENDIX C. STUDY QUALITY ASSESSMENT CRITERIA

Study, year	Adequate description of population*	Non-biased selection†	Low loss to followup‡	Adequate prognostic factor measurement§	Adequate outcome measurement‖	Method of validation
Amarasingham, 2010[24]	Yes	Unsure (appears to be consecutive series but does not explicitly state this)	Unsure (did not report follow-up)	Yes	Yes	Derived and validated in same population using cross-validation methodology (75% derivation, 25% validation repeated 1000 times)
Anderson, 1985[22]	No (good description of inclusion system but no description of overall demographics)	Yes	Unsure (did not report follow-up)	No (several prognostic factors not clearly described)	No, included interhospital transfers and did not exclude deaths	Different large cohort
Billings, 2007[25]	Partly	Yes	Unsure	Yes	Partly – unclear if transfers and elective readmissions were excluded.	Split sample in a large cohort
Bottle, 2006[12]	Yes	Yes	Yes	Partly – unsure how accurate geographic deprivation scores are	Partly – unclear if transfers and elective readmissions were excluded.	Split sample in a large cohort
Burns, 1991[58]	Yes	Yes	Yes	Yes	Partly – unlikely that readmissions to other hospitals were captured	Split sample in a small cohort
CMS model, AMI Krumholz 2008[16]	Yes	Yes	Unsure	Yes	Yes	Split sample in a large cohort
CMS model, CHF Krumholz, 2008[15]	Yes	Yes	Partly (they excluded the 11% of patients for whom incomplete information was available)	Yes	Yes	Split sample in a large cohort
CMS model, Pneumonia Krumholz, 2008[17]	Yes	Yes	Unsure	Yes	Yes	Split sample in a large cohort

Risk Prediction Models for Hospital Readmission: A Systematic Review

Study, year	Adequate description of population*	Non-biased selection†	Low loss to followup‡	Adequate prognostic factor measurement§	Adequate outcome measurement‖	Method of validation
Coleman, 2004[27]	Yes	Yes	Partly - use of Medicare data ensures good degree of f/u, but data on transfers to skilled nursing facilities from home not readily available	Yes	Partly - outcome was complicated care transitions which included admission to skilled nursing facility from home. Not clear that such transfers were reliably identified using available datasets	Different large cohorts
Evans, 1988[59]	Partly - inclusion criteria not well defined.	Unsure (probably consecutive series)	Unsure	Yes	Partly - outcome combined hospital readmissions, skilled nursing transfer from hospital, and stay longer than mean expected for DRG. It is unclear how valid the use of this combined measure is. Not clear that elective readmissions and transfers were excluded.	Split sample in a small cohort
Halfon, 2006[13]	Yes	Yes	Unsure	Yes	Yes	Split sample in a large cohort
Hammill 2011[18]	Yes	Yes	Unsure	Yes	Partly – 20% of registry patient files could not be linked to Medicare claims data and, therefore, is not included in outcome determination	Bootstrapping in large cohort
Hasan, 2009[31]	Yes	Partly - large # excluded because they did not complete intake interview, mostly because they were discharged before they could be interviewed. Sample therefore will be skewed towards longer LOS patients	Unsure - # completing 30 D f/u to gather self-report utilization data unclear	Yes	Partly - readmissions to non-index hospitalization based on self-report and therefore subject to recall bias. Elective readmissions were included	Split sample in a large cohort

Study, year	Adequate description of population*	Non-biased selection†	Low loss to followup‡	Adequate prognostic factor measurement§	Adequate outcome measurement‖	Method of validation
Holloway, 1990[53]	Partly (validation cohort not clearly described)	Yes	Yes	Yes	Yes	Split sample in a large cohort
Holman, 2005[14]	Yes	Yes	Yes	Partly - well-described methods, but administrative data only and comorbidity variables could have captured complications rather than comorbidities. No mention of effort to validate administrative data against chart review data.	Yes	Split sample in a large cohort
Howell, 2009[54]	Yes	Yes	Yes	Yes	Partly - unclear how transfers were handled	Split sample in a large cohort
Krumholz, 2000[30]	Yes	Yes	Unsure	Yes	Partly - readmissions from state-specific HCFA database - cross-state readmissions wouldn't be captured	Different large cohorts
Morrissey, 2003[28]	Yes	Yes	Unsure	Partly - data based on medical chart review, but unclear how well certain factors such as smoking history were documented in the medical record	Partly - readmissions to other facilities were not captured, but it was a rural area and there were few other options for care	Different small cohorts
Naessens, 1992[23]	Yes	Yes	Unsure	Yes	Yes	Jackknife approach using portions of large cohort
Novotny, 2008[33]	Partly - exclusion included life expectancy < 6 months but it is unclear how this was determined.	Partly - consecutive patients but large # not reached before discharge and large # refused participation, many because they did not feel well and this could have skewed sample.	Yes	Yes	Partly - not clear that elective readmissions were excluded	Moderate size validation cohort only (validation of a previously derived instrument)

Risk Prediction Models for Hospital Readmission: A Systematic Review

Study, year	Adequate description of population*	Non-biased selection†	Low loss to followup‡	Adequate prognostic factor measurement§	Adequate outcome measurement‖	Method of validation
PARR model Billings, 2006[26]	Partly	Yes	Unsure	Unsure	Partly - unclear if transfers and elective readmissions were excluded.	Split sample in a large cohort
Philbin, 1999[19]	Yes	Yes	Unsure (did not report % of patients with outcome available, mean "follow-up" 6.9 months)	Partly - calendar year readmissions used as outcome and f/u interval was not included as a covariate	Partly (used calendar year readmissions rather than 12 months follow-up period, making admissions later in year less applicable. And, cross-state readmissions not captured)	Split sample in a large cohort
PRA (original) Boult, 1993[32]	Yes	Yes	Partly (21.9% of patient records were not available through the end of 1988 and thus were excluded, but a selectively corrected two stage probit model no common influence between likelihood of missing data and readmission)	Yes	Yes	Split sample in a large cohort
PRA validation Allaudeen, 2011[34]	Yes	Partly - enrolled patients and provider participants over only a 5 week period	Partly - unclear how many patients were contacted successfully for self-report utilization measure	Yes	Yes	Validation of a previously derived instrument (PRA)
Silverstein, 2008[20]	Yes	Yes	Unsure (did not report)	Partly (comorbidities only assessed via discharge ICD-9 coding, not via actual measurement methods/scales)	Partly (only included readmission to Baylor MC, not to outside facilities)	Split sample in a large cohort
Smith Index (original) Smith 1985[55]	Yes	Yes	Yes	Yes	Yes	Split sample in a small cohort
Smith Index validation Smith 1988[56]	Yes	Yes	Unsure	Yes	Partly - a single center study and unclear how well readmissions to outside hospitals were captured	Validation of a previously derived instrument

Study, year	Adequate description of population*	Non-biased selection†	Low loss to followup‡	Adequate prognostic factor measurement§	Adequate outcome measurement‖	Method of validation
Smith Index validation Smith, 1996[57]	Partly - one of the criteria was expectation that pt would live > 3 months, but unclear how this was determined and how many pts were excluded for this reason	Partly - consecutive patients, but 20% could not be reached before discharge and another 20% declined to participate. Characteristics of these pts "were similar".	Unsure	Yes	Yes	Bootstrapping in a small cohort
Thomas, 1996[21]	No	Yes	Unsure	Partly - unclear how severity and complexity variables were calculated	Yes	different cohort (unsure of size)
van Walraven, 2010[29]	Yes	Yes	Yes, follow-up on 95.6% of population	Yes	Partly - outcome was self-report. Readmissions were considered unplanned if not arranged when patient had been discharged from index hospitalization.	Different large cohort

* Study describes inclusion criteria for selecting patients, and for enrolled patients describes duration and severity of symptoms, demographics (at least age), and setting (primary care vs. occupational vs. other).

† Study either reports enrolling (or attempting to enroll) a consecutive series of patients meeting inclusion criteria, or a random sample.

‡ Data for at least one outcome available for at least 80% of patients at 6 months or later of follow-up.

§ Study describes reproducible and appropriate methods for measuring prognostic factors.

‖ Study describes reproducible and appropriate methods to define and identify readmission; transfers and deaths during index hospitalization were excluded.